Arthritis Issues Resolved

Remedies, Dieting, and Exercise Programs

Refuge Victor

Table of content

Chapter 1

Arthritis (joint inflammation) and types

Joint inflammation is certainly not a solitary illness; the term alludes to joint agony or joint sickness, and there are more than 100 kinds of joint inflammation and related conditions. Individuals of any age, race, and gender live with joint pain, and it is the main source of handicap in the U.S. It's generally normal among ladies, and even though it's anything but a sickness of maturing, a few sorts of joint pain happen in more established individuals more than more youthful individuals.

Normal joint inflammation side effects incorporate expanding, torment, solidness, and lessened scope of movement in joints. Side effects differ from gentle to serious and may go back and forth. Some might remain about no different for a long time, however, side effects can likewise advance and deteriorate over the long run. Serious joint pain can bring about persistent torment, and trouble performing day-to-day exercises and make strolling and climbing steps agonizing and tiring.

Joint inflammation can likewise cause extremely durable joint changes. These might be apparent, for example, bumpy finger joints, yet frequently the harm should be visible just on X-beams. A few sorts of joint inflammation influence the heart, eyes, lungs, kidneys, and skin as well as the joints.

Kinds of Joint inflammation

Osteoarthritis

Osteoarthritis (OA) is by a wide margin the most well-known kind of joint inflammation. It can harm practically any joint yet basically happens in the hands, spine, hips, and knees. OA was once viewed as a mileage illness in which ligament — the defensive layer on the closures of bones — wore out following quite a while of purpose. Yet, with additional exploration, the pondering OA has changed. Specialists currently realize that OA is an infection of the entire joint, not simply the ligament. Bones in impacted joints become more fragile, the connective tissue that keeps the joint intact disintegrates and irritation harms the joint coating. Despite many years of conviction, irritation assumes a critical part in OA, similar and most different sorts of joint pain.

There's likewise a developing agreement that provocative OA is one of a few subtypes of osteoarthritis. Other subtypes incorporate OA-related to

Post-horrible wounds, for example, a torn upper leg tendon or break
Business-related harm from truly requesting a position, like cultivating and development
Way of life factors, including abundance weight, absence of activity, and less than stellar eating routine
Albeit the predominance of OA will in general increment with age, it's anything but an unavoidable piece of becoming older. You can assist with forestalling joint issues by remaining dynamic, keeping a solid weight, and restricting food sources that stir up irritation like red meat, profoundly handled food sources, and sugar. Better wagers? Berries, mixed greens, wild salmon, entire grains, and olive oil.

If you as of now have gentle to direct joint agony and firmness, ordinary actual work, hot and cold treatments, sensible utilization of over-the-counter painkillers and assistive gadgets might assist with dealing with your side effects.

At the point when joint side effects are serious, causing restricted portability and influencing personal satisfaction, you might need to examine a careful arrangement with your PCP.

Immune system Provocative Joint inflammation

A sound insusceptible framework is defensive. It creates irritation to clear diseases and recuperates wounds. In any case, in provocative joint inflammation, the resistant framework is overactive, going after sound tissue, and remembering joints for the spine, hands, and feet. In certain individuals, irritation becomes foundational, harming the eyes, skin, heart, and different organs. Many, however not a wide range of fiery joint pain are viewed as immune system illnesses because the resistant framework loses the capacity to recognize self from not-self and assaults the body it should secure.

Rheumatoid joint pain (RA) is the most widely recognized type of immune system provocative joint pain. Psoriatic joint inflammation (public service announcement) hub spondyloarthritis (axSpA), gout, and adolescent joint inflammation are more uncommon and can be more difficult to analyze.

It's not understood what causes provocative joint pain in each individual, however, the overall agreement is that something in the climate — an infection, stress, or smoking, for models — can set it in hereditarily inclined individuals. Ongoing The ongoingtion has additionally featured the complicated and basic job of stomach microorganisms in safe-related fiery sicknesses like RA and public service announcements.

The trillions of for the most part accommodating bugs that live in your stomach, skin, and mouth, aggregately called the microbiome, manage resistant cells all through the body and shape how the safe framework capabilities in different illnesses. At the point when these immense microbial networks escape funds receivable due to horrible eating routines, anti-toxin treatment, stress, or another variable, they may never again direct the safe reaction in a typical manner. This is believed to be one of the vital contributing variables to RA and other immune system-related incendiary circumstances.

With the immune system and provocative kinds of joint inflammation, early analysis and treatment are basic. Easing back sickness movement can help limit or forestall super durable joint harm as well as diminish torment and further develop capability and personal satisfaction. Reduction (characterized as practically zero sickness action) is consistently the objective, however low infection movement might be a more reasonable objective for certain individuals.

This is normally best accomplished with a blend of prescriptions and a solid way of life — customary activity, serene rest, quality food decisions, and less pressure. The prescription relies upon the kind of joint pain, the seriousness of side effects, and how well somebody answers a specific medication. For certain individuals, the main medication attempted may not be the best fit. What's more, some joint inflammation medications can make upsetting side impacts or lose their adequacy over the long haul. It might take a couple of attempts to track down the right drug.

Irresistible Joint pain

A bacterial, viral, or parasitic disease triggers irresistible joint pain. It typically begins when a disease from one more piece of the body goes to a joint, normally the knee. Side effects like enlarging, agony, and fever can be abrupt and extreme, yet treatment with anti-toxins or antifungals normally clears the contamination before long. Most popular contaminations are most recent for up to 14 days and disappear all alone. Certain individuals with irresistible joint pain might have to have their joint liquid depleted to eliminate tainted synovial liquid, decrease agony and aggravation, and forestall joint harm.

Gout (Metabolic Joint pain)

Metabolic or gouty joint pain — usually known as gout — results from the development in joints of difficult uric corrosive precious stones. These are a side-effect of the breakdown of purines — substances regularly tracked down in human cells and numerous food sources, particularly red meat, organ meats, a few shellfish, and liquor. Typically the body disposes of an abundance of uric corrosive, yet when it doesn't, it can collect in joints, causing unexpected and serious episodes of agony, particularly the enormous toe.

Nonetheless, the vast majority with high uric corrosive levels never foster gout and numerous gout patients have ordinary uric corrosive. An examination proposes that specific variables notwithstanding uric corrosive could set off gout. Potential offenders incorporate harm from OA, disturbances in the microbiome, and, surprisingly, white platelets in the liquid inside joints. Certain individuals experience just a single gout assault, or flare, and never have different side effects. They don't ordinarily need medicine. Individuals who have more than one gout flare or serious side effects are normally endorsed uric corrosive bringing down drugs. Those medications can make serious side impacts (and may not resolve the genuine issue), so as well as taking drugs, patients are encouraged to embrace a for the most part plant-based, low-purine diet, rich in natural products, vegetables, entire grains, olive oil, and low-purine fish.

Chapter 2
Symptoms and causes
The most widely recognized signs and side effects of joint inflammation include the joints. Contingent upon the kind of joint inflammation, signs, and side effects might include:

- Torment
- Firmness
- Enlarging
- Redness
- Diminished scope of movement

Causes
The two primary sorts of joint pain — osteoarthritis and rheumatoid joint pain — harm joints in various ways.

Osteoarthritis
The most well-known sort of joint pain, osteoarthritis, includes mileage harm to a joint's ligament — the hard, smooth covering on the finishes of bones where they structure a joint. Ligament pads the finishes of the bones and permits almost frictionless joint movement, yet enough harm can bring about bone crushing straightforwardly on bone, which causes torment and limited development. This mileage can happen over numerous years, or it tends to be rushed by a joint injury or disease.
Osteoarthritis additionally causes changes in the bones and disintegration of the connective tissues that append muscle to bone and keep the joint intact. On the off chance that the ligament in a joint is seriously harmed, the joint coating might become kindled and enlarged.

Rheumatoid joint pain
In rheumatoid joint pain, the body's resistant framework goes after the coating of the joint case, an extreme layer that encases every one of the joint parts. This coating (synovial film) becomes kindled and enlarged. The illness cycle can ultimately obliterate ligaments and bones inside the joint.

Risk factors for joint inflammation include:
Family ancestry. A few kinds of joint pain run in families, so you might be bound to foster joint pain on the off chance that your folks or kin have the problem.

Age. The gamble of many kinds of joint pain — including osteoarthritis, rheumatoid joint inflammation, and gout — increases with age.

Your sex. Ladies are more likely than men to foster rheumatoid joint inflammation, while a large portion of individuals who have gout, one more sort of joint pain, are men.

Past joint injury. Individuals who have harmed a joint, maybe while playing a game, are bound to foster joint inflammation in that joint ultimately.
Heftiness. Conveying an abundance of pounds puts weight on joints, especially your knees, hips, and spine. Individuals with heftiness have a higher gamble of creating joint pain.
Inconveniences

Extreme joint inflammation, especially if it influences your hands or arms, can make it challenging for you to do day-to-day undertakings. Joint inflammation of weight-bearing joints can hold you back from strolling easily or sitting upright. At times, they joined their arrangement and shape.

Chapter 3
Diagnosis, Treatment, and Remedies

Diagnosis
During the actual test, specialists take a look at your joints for expansion,
redness, and warmth. They'll likewise need to perceive how well you can
move your joints.

Lab tests
The investigation of various kinds of body liquids can assist with
pinpointing the sort of joint pain you might have. Liquids ordinarily
investigated incorporate blood, pee, and joint liquid. To get an example of a
joint liquid, specialists scrub and numb the region before embedding a
needle in the recuperates to pull out some liquid.
These kinds of tests can identify issues inside the joint that might be
causing your side effects. Models include:

X-beams. Utilizing low degrees of radiation to imagine bone, X-beams can
show ligament misfortune, bone harm, and bo,ne prods. X-beams may not
uncover early ligament harm, however, they are many times used to follow
the movement of thbecauseted tomography (CT). CT scanners take
X-beams from a wide range of points and join the data to make
cross-sectional perspectives on inner designs. CTs can imagine both bone
and the encompassing delicate tissues.

Attractive reverberation imaging (X-ray). Joining radio waves with areas of
strength for a field, X-ray can create more definite cross-sectional pictures
of delicate tissues like ligaments, ligaments, and tendons.

Ultrasound. This innovation utilizes high-recurrence sound waves,s to
picture delicate tissues, ligaments, and liquid-containing structures close,
to the joints (bursae). Ultrasound is additionally inclined in individual
simulating joint liquid or infusing drugs into the joint.

Treatment

Joint pain treatment centers have unsafe-related side effects and work on joint capability announcements have to attempt a few unique medicines, or blends of medicines, before you figure ouhout turns out best for you.

Prescriptions
The prescriptions used to treat joint pain differ contingent upon the kind of joint inflammation. Ordinarily utilized joint pain meds include:

NSAIDs. Nonsteroidal calming drugs (NSAIDs) can reduce the use of torment and lesroutinesitation. Models incorporate ibuprofen (Advil, Motrin IB, others) and naproxen sodium (Aleve). More grounded NSAIDs can cause stomach disturbance and may build your gamble of a coronary episode or stroke. NSA system-related accessible as creams or gels, which can be scoured on joints.
Counterirritants. A few assortments of creams and treatments contain menthol or capsaicin, the fixing that makes hot peppers fiery. Scouring these arrangements on the skin over your hurting joint might obstruct the transmission of torment signals from the actual joint.
Steroids. Corticosteroid prescriptions, like prednisone, decrease aggravation and torment and slow joint harm. Corticosteroids might be given as a pill or as an infusion into the difficult joint. Secondary effects might incorporate diminishing bones, weight gain, and diabetes.
Sickness adjusting antirheumatic drugs (DMARDs). These medications can slow the movement of rheumatoid joint inflammation, and save the joints and different tissues from extremely durable harm. Notwithstanding customary DMARDs, there are likewise biologic specialists and designated manufactured DMARDs. Incidental effects change however most DMARDs increment your gamble of contaminations.

Treatment
Active recuperation can be useful for certain kinds of joint pain. Activities can further the scope of movement and reinforce the muscles encompassing joints. At times, support might be justified.

Medical procedure

If moderate measures don't help, sp, specialists might recommend a medical procedure, for example,

Joint fix. In certain occasions, joint surfaces can be smoothed or realigned to lessen torment and further develop elop capability. These kinds of strategies can frequently be performed
arthroscopically — through little entry points over the joint.

Joint substitution. This system eliminates the harmed joint and replaces it with a counterfeit one. The joints most normally supplanted are the hips and knees.

Joint combination. This method is frequently utilized for more modest joints, like those in the wrist, lower leg, and fingers. It eliminates the finishes of the two bones in the joint and afterward locks those closures together until they mend into one unbending unit.

As a rule, joint pain side effects can be decreased with the accompanying measures:

Weight reduction. An overabundance of weight puts additional weight on weight-bearing joints. Getting in shape might expand your portability and cause future joint injury.

Work out. Ordinary activity can assist with keeping joints adaptable. Swimming and water vigorous exercise might be great decisions because the lightness of the water lessens the weight on weight-bearing joints.

Intensity and cold. Warming cushions or ice packs might assist with easing joint inflammation torment.

Assistive gadgets. Utilizing sticks, shoe embeds, walkers, raised latrine seats, and other assistive gadgets can assist with safeguarding joints and working on your capacity to perform everyday assignments.

Many individuals utilize elective solutions for joint inflammation, however, there is minimal dependable proof to help the utilization of a significant number of these drugs ms. The most encouraging elective solutions for joint pain include:

Needle therapy. Treatment utilizes products and needles with an explicit focus on the skin to lessen many sorts of agony, including that brought about by certain kinds of joint inflammation.

Glucosamine. Even though study results have been blended, a few investigations have discovered that glucosamine works no better compared to fake treatment. Be that as it may, glucosamine and the fake treatment both eased osteoarthritis torment better compared to taking
nothing, especially in individuals who have moderate to extreme agony from knee osteoarthritis.

Chondroitin. Chondroitin might give humble help with discomfort from osteoarthritis, even though study results are blended.

Fish oil. A few primer investigations have discovered that fish oil enhancements might lessen the side effects of certain sorts of joint pain. Fish oil can disrupt prescriptions, so check with your primary care physician first.

Yoga and kendo. The sluggish, extending developments related to yoga and kendo may assist with winning on joint adaptability and scope of movement.

Rub. Light stroking and plying of muscles might increment blood stream and warm impact the d joints, briefly easing torment. Ensure your back rub specialist realizes which joints are impacted by joint inflammation.

Getting ready for your arrangement

While you could initially examine your side effects with your family specialist, the person might allude to an in-the-specialist treatment of joint issues (rheumatologist) for additional assessment.

What you can do ligaments your arrangement, make a rundown that incorporates:

- Point-by-point portrayals of your side effects
- Data about clinical issues you've had before
- Data about the clinical issues of your folks or kin
- Every one of the drugs and dietary enhancements you take
- Questions you need to ask the specialist
- What's in store from your primary care physician

Your, primary care physician might pose a portion of the accompalikelyquiries:
- When did your side effects begin? Improve or more terrible?
- Which joints are difficult?
- Do you have a family background of joint torment?

Chapter 4

Exercise and Dieting

Might it be said that you are eased back or hampered by the agony of joint inflammation? An expected 54.4 million U.S. grown-ups (23%) have a specialist-of-analyzed joint pain, and this number is projected to ascend to 78.4 million in the following 20 years. The rates analyzed fluctuate generally by area, with 17% in Hawaii and up to 43 percent in states. Regions with higher rates have a higher populace of more seasoned day-to-day and stoutness, both gamble factors for joint inflammation. There are a few sorts of joint inflammation, yet for this article, osteoarthritis and rheumatoid joint pain, two of the most well-known structures, will be examined.

Osteoarthritis

Osteoarthritis (OA) is the most well-known type of joint pain, influencing more than 30 million individuals in the US. OA is the quickest-developing reason for handicaps around the world. It is in some cases called degenerative joint sickness or "mileage" joint pain. It most often happens in the hands, hips, and knees. With OA, the ligament, or the dangerous tissue that covers the closures of bones in a joint, starts to separate. Before the ligament, the bones rub together, causing torment and firmness. OA can likewise cause expansion and bring about inability. Family ancestry and joint injury are likewise risk factors for OA.

Active work and OA

Exercise and routine day-to-day active work are suggested as endured, as they frequently work on joint agony and portability. Counsel your primary care physician initially; 150 minutes of moderate actual work each week is suggested for grown-ups, incorporating those with OA. Strolling, trekking, and swimming are ordinarily all around endured. Yoga and judo further develop equilibrium and adaptability, while yoga likewise further develops strength. These activities assist with keeping up with our capacity to perform exercises of day-to-day living, for example, lifting food and strolling up advances, in ligaments, diminishing handicap and agony. Customary active work further develops mindset, diminishes the risk of despondency, and ligaments, and de-liquid-containing Lewis assists with weight reduction and weight control, which is critical for those with OA, as stoutness is normal and further corrupts joints and debilitates portability.

Sustenance Proposals for OA
As far as sustenance research, the heft of studies have checked out individual supplements or food varieties and their job with aggravation. Nonetheless, this approach has numerous limits since our eating regimen is comprised of numerous food sources, with numerous singular food parts and connections.

Follow a Mediterranean eating design - An exceptionally huge, cross-sectional investigation of 4,470 grown-ups with OA broke down diet scores contrasted with the Mediterranean eating regimen (high measures of vegetables, natural products, entire grains, fish, olive oil, and nuts; restricted a meat, poultry, and full-fat dairy). Higher Mediterranean eating routine scores were essentially connected with superior personal satisfaction and less torment, solidness, incapacity, and melancholy. Starting around 2015, this eating design has been suggested by the Dietary Rules for Americans for everybody.
Get in shape if overweight - Studies show even a 5 percent weight reduction (regularly 10 to 12 pounds) will assist with lessening agony and increment portability. Shedding pounds additionally lessens irritation. Following a Mediterranean eating example might assist with controlling weight, even though it's anything but a proper weight reduction diet. Ask your doctor for a reference to an enrolled dietitian nutritionist for the best individual suggestions.

Omega-3 Unsaturated fats - A few examinations in the previous ten years have shown the useful impacts of omega-3 unsaturated fats and diminishing knee ligament misfortune and irritation. Greasy fish, like salmon, fish, and trout, are suggested no less than two times per week.

Decrease admission of immersed fats - A few investigations show a relationship between high blood cholesterol levels and ligament corruption.

Different examinations embroil soaked fat in expanding irritation. A different report shows a bigger gamble for OA and rheumatoid joint pain with expanded utilization of aggregate and handled meats in the Unified Realm. Devour red meats and full-fat dairy food varieties less than one to two times each week.

Vitamin D - Studies have shown low vitamin D blood levels are firmly connected with OA movement and ligament misfortune. Our bodies can make vitamin D with 20 minutes of face and arm sun openness. Nonetheless, polishing off The joints with D-strengthened low-fat milk, yogurt, or enhancements of 25 mcg each day has been suggested for predictable blood vitamin D levels.

Vitamin K - When lacking, one enormous review showed more knee OA and ligament sores since vitamin K is significant in ligament digestion. Green verdant vegetables are phenomenal sources and ought to be consumed frequently.

Rheumatoid joint pain
Rheumatoid joint pain (RA) is the most well-known type of immune system joint inflammation. It influences more than 1.3 million Americans. Around 75% of RA patients are ladies, most frequently analyzed between age 30 and 50. It is caused when the body's invulnerable framework isn't working as expected and erroneously goes after the joint tissues. RA because of the wrist and little joints of the tend and feet, fevers, and exhaustion. Drawn-out morning solidness can be one sign of RA.

Exercise and Sustenance Proposals for RA
Exercise and nourishment suggestions for RA are equivalent to those talked about above for OA since side effects are comparative for solidness, agony, and working portability. Be that as it may, since RA is an immune system problem, there are a few extra eating routine proposals:

Fiber -, C-responsive protein (CRP) in the blood is a marker of irritation related to RA. A few investigations have revealed that a high-fiber diet decreases CRP levels. Oats, brown and wild rice, beans, grain, and quinoa are brilliant wellsprings of entire grains and fiber. Nuts, seeds, and entire leafy foods are additionally great wellsprings of fiber.

Probiotics - The stomach's microscopic organisms are changed with RA, and it is guessed some food parts, similar to proteins, are mistakenly going through the gastrointestinal film and causing aggravation as our bodies assault it. Probiotics, or microbes from food like yogurt or enhancements that are great for the stomach, have been displayed in certain examinations to assist with RA side effects. More examinations are required; counsel a doctor before taking any even though berry juice - A few examinations have shown that 2 cups of cranberry squeeze every day gives calming and cell reinforcement impacts, diminishing irritation in RA. More investigations are required.

High-fructose corn syrup improved (HFCS) sodas - A couple of studies show a relationship with RA. Those polishing off Hot Sodas at least five times each week were multiple times bound to have RA.

Doubtful Food and Diet Solutions for Joint Inflammation
As per the Joint Inflammation Establishment, coming up next are not experimentally upheld; consequently, they are not prescribed to alleviate joint inflammation side effects: Taking or following:

- Gelatin and collagen,
- Gelatin,
- Soluble eating routine,
- Juice vinegar,
- Espresso,
- Crude eating regime redfern-drenched rai

Staying away from:
- Citrus food varieties (because of acridity),
- Dairy (attempt skim or low fat, or lactose-free if lactose prejudiced),

- Nightshade Vegetables Int-by-pointes, potatoes, eggplants, and peppers (these contain the synthetic solanine, which some fault for joint inflammation torment).

While the quantity of individuals with joint pain is developing, the requirement for exact data on sustenance and exercise is also. Following a solid eating regimen and actual work suggestions is fundamental for treatment, keeping up with personal satisfaction, and improving with counteraction. Continuously counsel your medical care supplier before starting any new activity or diet change.

A definitive Joint inflammation Diet
Gain which food sources from the Mediterranean eating routine can assist with battling irritation brought about by joint pain.

Perhaps of the most widely recognized question individuals with joint inflammation ask is, "Is there an exceptional joint inflammation diet?" While there's no marvel diet for joint pain, numerous food sources can assist with battling irritation and work on joint torment and different side effects.

First of all, an eating routine wealthy in entire food sources, including organic products, vegetables, fish, nuts and beans, however low handled food sources and soaked fat, isn't just perfect for generally wellbeing, yet can likewise assist with overseeing illness action. Assuming this exhortation sounds recognizable, this is on the grounds that these are the standards of the Mediterranean eating routine, which is much of the time promoted for its calming and infection battling powers.

Mediterranean Eating routine
Studies affirm that eating food sources generally a piece of the Mediterranean eating regimen have the accompanying advantages:
- Lower pulse
- Safeguard against ongoing circumstances, going from malignant growth to stroke
- Help joint pain by controlling irritation
- Benefit your joints as well as your heart

- Lead to weight reduction, which can decrease joint agony

Here are key food varieties from the Mediterranean eating regimen and for what reason they're so really great for joint wellbeing. Track down more data to oversee torment with our aggravation assets.

Fish
The amount: Wellbeing specialists like the American Heart Affiliation and the Institute of Sustenance and Dietetics prescribe three to four ounces of fish, two times per week. Joint pain specialists guarantee more is better.
Why: A few sorts of fish are great wellsprings of irritation battling omega-3 unsaturated fats. One review found the individuals who had the most noteworthy utilization of omega-3s had lower levels of two provocative proteins: C-responsive protein (CRP) and interleukin-6. All the more as of late, scientists have shown that taking fish oil supplements diminishes joint enlarging and torment, term of morning firmness and illness action among individuals who have rheumatoid joint pain (RA).
Best sources: Salmon, fish, sardines, herring, anchovies, scallops and other cold-water fish. Can't stand fish? Take an enhancement. Concentrates on show that taking 600 to 1,000 mg of fish oil day to day facilitates joint firmness, delicacy, agony and expanding.

Nuts and Seeds
The amount: Eat 1.5 ounces of nuts day to day (one ounce is about a modest bunch).
Why: "Different examinations affirm the job of nuts in a calming diet," makes sense of José M. Ordovás, PhD, head of nourishment and genomics at the Jean Mayer USDA Human Sustenance Exploration Center on Maturing at Tufts College in Boston. One investigation discovered that north of a 15-year time span, people who consumed the most nuts had a 51% lower hazard of biting the dust from a provocative infection (like RA) contrasted with the individuals who ate the least nuts. Another investigation discovered that subjects with lower levels of vitamin B6 — saw as in many nuts — had more significant levels of provocative markers.

All the more uplifting news: Nuts are jam-loaded with irritation battling monounsaturated fat. What's more, however they're generally high in fat and calories, concentrates on show noshing on nuts advances weight reduction in light of the fact that their protein, fiber and monounsaturated fats are satisfying. "Simply remember that more isn't generally better," says Ordovás.
Best sources: Pecans, pine nuts, pistachios and almonds.

Organic products and Vegetables
The amount: Hold back nothing more servings day to day (one serving rises to one cup of most veggies or natural product or two cups of crude salad greens).
Why: Products of the soil are stacked with cancer prevention agents. These strong synthetic substances go about as the body's normal protection framework, assisting with killing shaky particles called free revolutionaries that can harm cells. Research has shown that anthocyanins found in cherries and other red and purple natural products like strawberries, raspberries, blueberries and blackberries make a mitigating difference.
All the more uplifting news: Citrus organic products — like oranges, grapefruits and limes — are plentiful in L-ascorbic acid. Research shows getting the perfect proportion of that nutrient guides in forestalling provocative joint pain and keeping up with sound joints. Other exploration proposes eating vitamin K-rich veggies like broccoli, spinach, lettuce, kale and cabbage decisively diminishes provocative markers in the blood.
Best sources: Bright foods grown from the ground — the hazier or more splendid the variety, the more cell reinforcements it has. Great ones incorporate blueberries, cherries, spinach, kale and broccoli.

Olive Oil
The amount: A few tablespoons everyday.
Why: Olive oil is stacked with heart-sound fats, as well as oleocanthal, which has properties like nonsteroidal mitigating drugs (NSAIDs). "Oleocanthal hinders movement of COX chemicals, with a pharmacological activity like ibuprofen," says Ordovás. Repressing these compounds hoses the body's fiery cycles and decreases torment responsiveness.

Best sources: Additional virgin olive oil goes through less refining and handling, so it holds a bigger number of supplements than standard assortments. Furthermore, it's not by any means the only oil with medical advantages. Avocado and safflower oils have shown cholesterol-bringing down properties, while pecan oil has multiple times the omega-3s that olive oil has.

Beans
The amount: Around one cup, two times per week (or more).
Why: Beans are stacked with fiber and phytonutrients, which assist with bringing down CRP, a sign of aggravation tracked down in the blood. At significant levels, CRP could show anything from contamination to RA. In a review researchers broke down the supplement content of 10 normal bean assortments and recognized a large group of cell reinforcement and calming compounds. Beans are additionally a superb and economical wellspring of protein and have around 15 grams for every cup, which is significant for muscle wellbeing.
Best sources: Little red beans, red kidney beans and pinto beans rank among the U.S. Branch of Horticulture's main four cell reinforcement containing food sources (wild blueberries take the number 2 spot).

Entire Grains
The amount: Eat a sum of six ounces of grains each day; no less than three of which ought to come from entire grains. One ounce of entire grain would be equivalent to ½ cup cooked earthy colored rice or one cut of entire wheat bread.
Why: Entire grains contain a lot of filling fiber — which can assist you with keeping a sound weight. A few examinations have likewise demonstrated the way that fiber and fiber-rich food varieties can bring down blood levels of CRP, an incendiary marker.
Best sources: Eat food varieties made with the whole grain portion, similar to entire wheat flour, cereal, bulgur, earthy colored rice and quinoa. Certain individuals should be cautious about which entire grains they eat. Gluten — a protein tracked down in wheat and different grains — has been connected to irritation for individuals with celiac illness (Cd) or gluten responsiveness.

Nightshade Vegetables

Why: Nightshade vegetables, including eggplant, tomatoes, red chime peppers and potatoes, are sickness battling forces to be reckoned with that brag greatest sustenance for insignificant calories.

What difference would it make: They likewise contain solanine, a synthetic that has been marked the offender in joint pain torment. There's no logical proof to propose that nightshades trigger joint pain flares.

Test it: A few specialists accept these vegetables contain an intense supplement blend that hinders joint inflammation torment. Be that as it may, many individuals really do report side effect alleviation when they stay away from nightshade vegetables. In this way, assuming that you notice that your joint pain torment flares in the wake of eating them, consider killing all nightshade vegetables from your eating routine so that half a month might check whether it has an effect. Then, at that point, gradually add them back into your eating regimen to check whether side effects deteriorate or remain something similar.